P9-EFJ-087

TREAT YOUR OWN NECK

TREAT
YOUR OWN NECK

By
ROBIN McKENZIE, O.B.E., F.C.S.P., F.N.Z.S.P. (Hon) DIP. M.T.

SPINAL PUBLICATIONS NEW ZEALAND LTD.

Spinal Publications
Postal address: P.O. Box 93, Waikanae, New Zealand.

© Robin McKenzie 1983.

ISBN 0 473 00209 4

First Published 1983.
Reprinted October, 1983   December, 1986
          January, 1984   October, 1987
          April, 1984   August, 1988
          November, 1984   October, 1989
          March, 1985   August, 1990
          December, 1985   June, 1991
          July, 1986   May, 1992

Photography:
John Tristram, Juniper Films,
27A Roosevelt Street, Levin, New Zealand.

ACKNOWLEDGEMENT

My special thanks for assistance in the production of this book, must go to Paula Van Wijmen. Paula edited and corrected my manuscripts and helped in no small way in clarifying the material contained within.

Paula received her physiotherapy training in The Netherlands where she graduated in physiotherapy in 1967. She worked in Canada for eight years and since that time has been in full time private practice in New Zealand where she assisted in my clinic in the city of Wellington. In 1979 Paula received a Diploma in Manipulative Therapy, from the New Zealand Manipulative Therapists Association.

Paula is now mainly involved in the education of health professionals both in New Zealand and overseas.

Robin McKenzie.

ABOUT THE AUTHOR

Robin McKenzie was born in Auckland, New Zealand, in 1931. After attending Wairarapa College he enrolled in the New Zealand School of Physiotherapy, from which he graduated in 1952. He commenced his private practice in Wellington, New Zealand in 1953, and soon developed special interest in the treatment of spinal problems.

During the sixties Robin McKenzie developed his own examination and treatment methods and since then he has become recognised internationally as an authority on the diagnosis and treatment of low back pain. He has lectured extensively in North America, Europe, Australia and New Zealand where his methods for treating low back pain are now widely practised. He has published in the *New Zealand Medical Journal* and is the author of four books: *Treat Your Own Back, Treat Your Own Neck* (which have been translated into Spanish, Dutch, French, German, Chinese and Italian), *The Lumbar Spine, Mechanical Diagnosis and Therapy,* and *The Cervical and Thoracic Spine, Mechanical Diagnosis and Therapy.*

Robin McKenzie is a member of the New Zealand Manipulative Therapists Association. He is a consultant and lecturer to the Orthopaedic Physical Therapy Programme at the Kaiser Permanente Medical Centre in Hayward, California, and a member of the Editorial Board for the *North American Journal of Orthopaedic Physical Therapy and Sports Medicine.*

His contributions to the understanding and treatment of spinal problems have been recognised both in New Zealand and internationally. In 1982 he was made an Honorary Life Member of the American Physical Therapy Association, *in recognition of distinguished and meritorious service to the art and science of physical therapy and to the welfare of mankind.* In 1983 he was elected to membership of the International Society for the Study of the Lumbar Spine. In 1984 he was made a Fellow of the American Back Society, and in 1985 he was awarded an Honorary Fellowship of the New Zealand Society of Physiotherapists.

CONTENTS

Acknowledgement   5

CHAPTER 1   Introduction   9

2   The neck or cervical spine   12

3   Common causes of neck pain   23

4   Exercises   38

5   When to apply the exercises   56

6   General instructions   61

7   Summary   63

CHAPTER 1

INTRODUCTION

Neck problems are referred to in different ways such as arthritis in the neck, spondylosis of the neck, rheumatism, fibrositis, slipped disc; or, when it concerns pain extending into the arm, neuritis and neuralgia.

Most of us suffer at some time during our life from pain in the region of the neck, or pain arising from the neck which is felt across the shoulders, in the shoulder blade, the upper or lower arm. Pain coming from the neck can also be felt in the hand and symptoms such as pins and needles or numbness can be experienced in the fingers. Some people are troubled by headaches, the cause of which can be traced to problems in the neck.

Usually these aches and pain occur intermittently — that is, there are times in the day or there are days that no pain is felt. The symptoms may appear mysteriously, often for no apparent reason, and just as mysteriously they disappear. These aches and pains may also occur constantly — that is, pain to some degree or other is felt at all times. People who have pain all of the time are frequently forced to take pills. It is uncommon for these people to have to stop work, although this occasionally happens. More often the pain simply makes their life miserable and they have to reduce their activities in order to keep the discomfort at a moderate level. Neck problems can thus affect our lifestyle.

If you have problems of this nature, you may already have discovered that the symptoms can last sometimes for months or even years. Or you may have found out that treatments are often able to stop your pain, but the pain returns at some time later to affect you once more. You may be reading this book because you have persistent pains that have not disappeared, despite the fact that you may have received the best of treatment. Whatever the situation, you most likely will realise that many of the treatments, dispensed by doctors, physiotherapists and chiropractors, are prescribed for your present symptoms and are not directed at preventing future problems. Time and again you may have to seek assistance to get relief from your neck pain. How good it would be if you were able to apply treatment to yourself whenever pain were to make itself felt. Better still, how good it would be if you were able to apply a system of treatment to yourself that would prevent the onset of pain.

Only in the past ten to fifteen years have the methods been discovered that enable us to learn to manage our own spinal problems. Unfortunately, this information has not been disseminated widely until recently for, like many developments within medicine, new ideas must be seen to be effective before they can be supported. The methods I am going to describe to you have been used by doctors and physiotherapists in many parts of the world since the early 1970's and generally their patients are achieving the same satisfactory results.

One of the main points of this book is that the management of your neck is *your* responsibility. If, for some reason or other, *you* have developed neck problems, then *you* must learn how to deal with the present symptoms and how to prevent future problems. Self-treatment will be more effective in the long term management of your neck pain than any other form of treatment.

This book is not meant for you, at least not at this stage, if you have developed neck pain for the first time. In that case you should consult your doctor who will look into your neck problems from the various medical angles. When appropriate he will refer you to a manipulative therapist for treatment, and more important, for advice and instructions on the prevention of further neck problems. You should also seek advice if there are complications to your neck problems, for example if you have severe and stabbing pains, if your head is pulled off-centre or if you have severe unabating headaches.

A manipulative therapist is a physiotherapist specialised in the treatment of disturbances in the musculo-skeletal system. In the U.S.A. such a therapist is known as an orthopaedic physical therapist.

Finally, this book will help only eighty percent of the people with neck pain; it is meant for those with straight forward mechanical problems. Hopefully you fall into this category and will find the information clear and useful.

CHAPTER 2

THE NECK OR CERVICAL SPINE

THE SPINE

Let us look at the human backbone (*Fig. 2:1*), the spine or spinal column. In the area of the neck the spine consists of seven bones, the vertebrae, which rest upon one another similarly to a stack of cotton spools. Each vertebra has a solid part in front, called the vertebral body, and a hole in the back (*Fig. 2:2*). When lined up as the spinal column, these holes form the spinal canal. This canal serves as a protected passageway for the spinal cord, the bundle of nerves which extends from head to pelvis.

Separating the vertebrae are special cartilages, called the discs. These are located between the vertebral bodies just in front of the spinal cord (*Fig. 2:2*). Each disc consists of a soft fluid centre part, the nucleus, which is surrounded and held together by a cartilage ring, the annulus or annular ligament. The discs are similar to rubber washers and act as shock absorbers. They are able to alter their shape, thus allowing movement of one vertebra on another and of the neck as a whole.

The vertebrae and discs are linked up by a series of joints to form the cervical spine or neck. Each joint is held together by its surrounding soft tissues — that is, a capsule reinforced by ligaments. Muscles lie over one or more joints of the neck and may extend upwards to the head or downwards to the trunk. At both ends each muscle changes into a tendon by which it attaches itself to different bones. When a muscle contracts it causes movement in one or more joints.

Between each two vertebrae there is a small opening on either side through which a nerve leaves the spinal canal, the right and left spinal nerve (*Fig. 2:3*). Amongst other tasks the spinal nerves supply our muscles with power and our skin with sensation. The nerves are really part of our alarm system: pain is the warning that some structure is about to be damaged or has already sustained some damage.

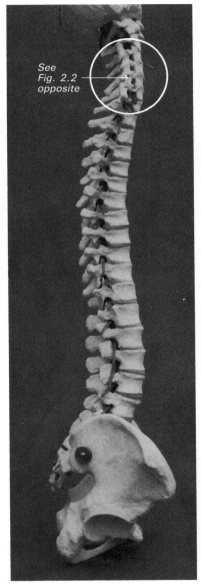

See
Fig. 2.2
opposite

Fig. 2:1
The spine or spinal column,
facing right.

Fig. 2:2
Two cervical vertebrae with
disc between.

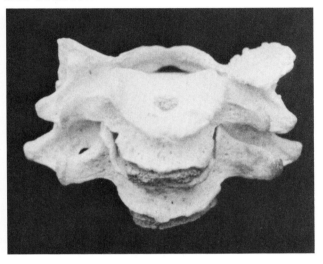

Fig. 2:3
Vertebrae and emerging nerve.

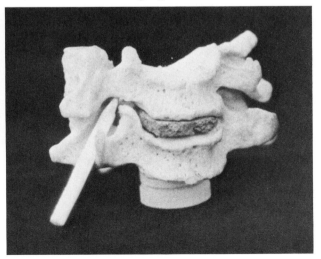

FUNCTIONS OF THE CERVICAL SPINE

On top of this complex of bones and washers rests the head which contains our computer system, the brain, and the important sensors associated with it such as the eyes, ears, nose and mouth. Together the vertebrae, discs and head form a series of flexible joints which allow the head to turn almost 180 degrees from one side to the other, to look up and down, and to bend sideways. In addition the head can adopt many positions that are combinations of the movements mentioned above.

The main functions of the cervical spine are to support the head, allow it to move in many directions and adjust its position in fine degrees in order to assist the working of the sensors; and to provide a protected passageway for the bundle of nerves that extends from the brain to the sacrum, the tail end of the spine.

The neck has a high flexibility due to the specially designed structure of the joints, in particular those between the uppermost vertebrae and the head. Its flexibility is further increased because in this area no bony structures are attached to the spine. Thus, the neck can move relatively more freely than the rest of the spine where movements are restricted by ribcage and pelvis. On the other hand, because the neck is not surrounded and protected by other structures, it is also more vulnerable than the rest of the spine when subjected to strains. The very flexibility, so helpful and necessary for everyday living, is also the cause of many of our problems. The wide range of movement of the neck exposes it to an equally wide range of stresses and strains.

NATURAL POSTURE

The side view of the human body (*Fig. 2:4*) shows that there is a small inward curve in the neck just above the shoulder girdle. This is called the cervical lordosis. It is this curve in the spine that concerns us mainly in this book.

When standing upright the head should be carried directly above the shoulder girdle, thus forming a small but visible cervical lordosis. (*Fig. 2:4*) Due to postural neglect people can often be seen to carry the head in front of their body with their chin poking forward. (*Fig. 2:5*) Now the cervical lordosis is altered in shape and distorted. In this position the joints of the lower neck are relatively bent forwards or flexed, whereas those between the upper part of the neck and the head are bent backwards or extended. This is called the protruded head posture (*Fig. 2:5*) and, if present often and long enough, neck problems may develop.

Fig. 2:4
Side view of human body with good posture.

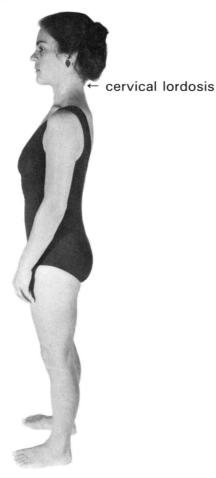

← cervical lordosis

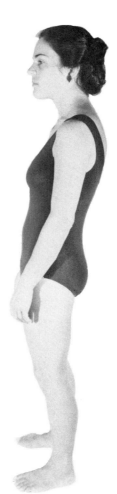

Fig. 2:5
Bad posture.

WHY NECK PAIN

Mechanical pain occurs when the joint between two bones has been placed in a position that overstretches the surrounding soft tissues. This is true for mechanical pain in any joint of the body, but in the spine there are additional factors. Here the tissues that surround the joints between the vertebrae, in particular the ligaments, are also responsible for supporting the soft discs that separate the vertebrae. They hold the discs in an enclosed compartment and help to form a shock absorbing mechanism.

Pain of mechanical origin may arise in the neck for the following reasons. The ligaments and other soft tissues which hold the vertebrae together can simply be overstretched without further damage. Overstretching may be caused by an outside force placing a sudden severe strain on the neck, for example due to an accident or during contact sport. This type of stress cannot easily be avoided as it occurs unexpectedly and takes a person unawares. More often overstretching is caused by postural stresses which place less severe strains on the neck over a longer time period. This type of stress is exerted *by ourselves on our own neck* and can easily be influenced. Here lies our main responsibility in the self-treatment and prevention of neck pain.

Complications arise when overstretching of soft tissues leads to actual tissue damage. It is often thought that neck pain is caused by strained muscles. Muscles, which are the source of power and cause movement, can indeed be overstretched and injured. This requires a considerable amount of external force and does not happen all that often. Moreover, muscles usually heal rapidly and seldom cause pain lasting for more than a week or two. On the other hand, whenever the impact of the injuring force is severe enough to affect muscles, the underlying soft tissues such as capsule and ligaments will be damaged as well. In fact, usually these are damaged long before the muscles. When these tissues heal they may form scar tissues, become less elastic and shorten. At this stage even normal movements may stretch the scars in these shortened structures and produce pain. Unless appropriate exercises are performed to gradually stretch and lengthen these structures and restore their normal flexibility, they may become a continuous source of neck pain or headaches.

Complications of another nature arise when the ligaments surrounding the disc are injured to such an extent that the disc loses its ability to absorb shock and its outer wall becomes weakened. This allows the soft inside of the disc to bulge outwards and, in extreme cases, to burst through the outer ligament, which may cause serious problems. When the disc bulge protrudes far enough backwards it may press painfully on a spinal nerve. This may cause some of the pains felt well away from the source of the trouble, for example in the arm or hand.

Due to this bulging the disc may become severely distorted and prevent the vertebrae from lining up properly during movement. In this case some movements may be blocked partially or completely and forcing of these movements causes severe pain. This is the reason that in some people the head can only be held in an off-centre position. Those of you, who experience a sudden onset of pain and following this are unable to move the head normally, may have some bulging of the soft disc material. This need not be a cause for alarm. The movements, described in this book, are carefully designed to reduce any disturbance of this nature.

POSTURAL STRESSES

The most common form of neck pain is caused by overstretching of ligaments due to postural stresses. This may occur when sitting with poor posture for a long time (*Fig. 2:6*); when lying or sleeping overnight with the head in an awkward position (*Fig. 2:7 and 2:7a*) and when working in strained positions (*Fig. 2:8*).

Of all these postural stresses the poor sitting posture — that is, sitting with the head protruded — is by far the one most often at fault. Poor posture in itself may produce neck pain. But, once neck problems have developed, poor posture will frequently make them worse and always perpetuate them.

The main theme of this chapter is that pain of postural origin will not occur, if you avoid prolonged overstretching. Should pain develop, then there are certain movements you can perform in order to stop that pain. You should not have to seek assistance whenever postural pain arises.

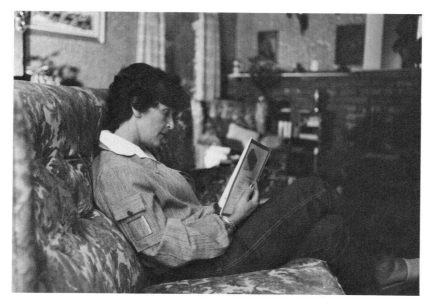

Fig. 2:6
Bad sitting position.

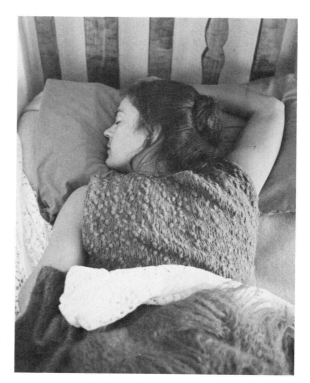

Fig. 2:7
Bad sleeping posture.

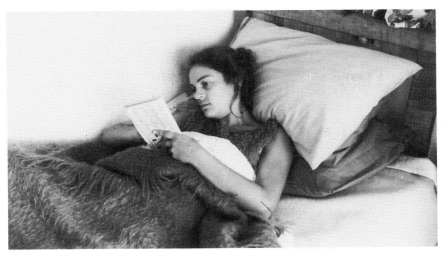

Fig. 2:7(a)
Bad lying posture.

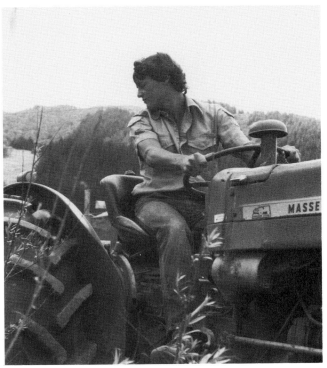

Fig. 2:8
Strained working
position.

WHERE IS THE PAIN FELT

The sites of pain caused by neck problems vary from one person to another. In a first attack pain is usually felt at or near the base of the neck, in the centre (*Fig. 2:9*) or just to one side (*Fig. 2:10*). Usually the pain subsides within a few days. In subsequent attacks pain may reach across both shoulders (*Fig. 2:11*), to the top of one shoulder or the shoulder blade (*Fig. 2:12*); and later still to the outside or back of the upper arm as far as the elbow (*Fig. 2:13*); or it may extend below the elbow to the wrist or hand and pins and needles or numbness may be felt in the fingers (*Fig. 2:14*). Some people experience headaches as a result of neck problems. Often these headaches are felt at the top of the neck and the base and back of the head, on one or both sides (*Fig. 2:15*); but they can also spread from the back of the head over the top of the head to above or behind the eye, again on one or both sides (*Fig. 2:16*).

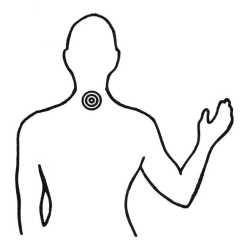

Fig. 2:9

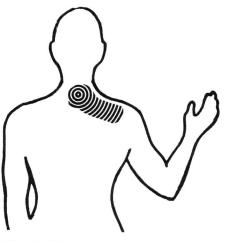

Fig. 2:10

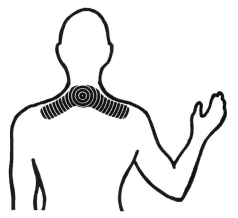

Fig. 2:11

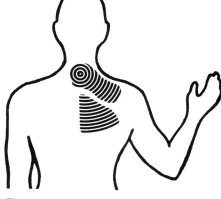

Fig. 2:12

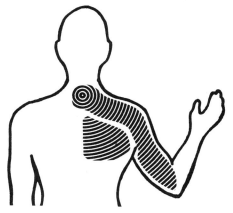

Fig. 2:13

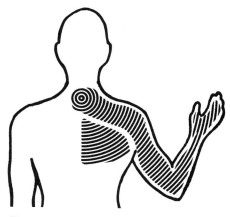

Fig. 2:14

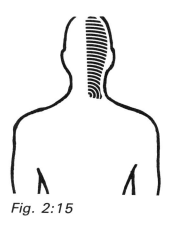

Fig. 2:15

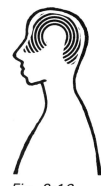

Fig. 2:16

21

WHO CAN PERFORM SELF-TREATMENT

There are only a few people who will not benefit from the advice given in this book. Nearly everyone can commence the exercise programme, provided the recommended precautions are taken. Once you have started the exercises, carefully watch your pain pattern. If your pains are getting progressively worse, and remain worse the following day, you should seek advice from your doctor or manipulative therapist.

In any of the following situations you should not commence the exercise programme without first consulting your doctor or manipulative therapist:

If you have pain near or at the wrist or hand and experience sensations of pins and needles or numbness in the fingers.

If you have developed neck problems following a recent, severe accident.

If you have developed headaches recently. In this case your eyes or spectacles may need to be checked out.

If you experience severe headaches which have come on for no apparent reason, never let off and are gradually getting worse.

If you have severe episodic headaches which are accompanied by nausea and dizziness.

CHAPTER 3
COMMON CAUSES OF NECK PAIN

1. Sitting for Prolonged Periods

When we are moving about, especially when walking briskly, we assume a fairly upright posture. The head is retracted and held directly over the vertebral column and consequently receives the maximum support possible. When we sit and relax in a chair, (*Fig. 3:1*) the head and neck slowly protrude because the muscles that support them become tired. As the muscles tire they relax and so we lose the main support for a good posture. The result is the protruded head posture (*Fig. 3:1a*). This posture can be seen around us every day. It is not present during infancy, but develops from mid-teens onwards. We are not really designed to sit for six to eight hours daily, perhaps six days a week.

Fig. 3:1
Bad sitting posture.

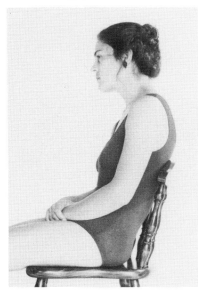

Fig. 3:1(a)
Protruded head posture.

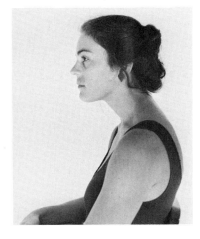

When the protruded head posture is maintained long enough, it causes overstretching of ligaments. Thus pain will arise *in certain positions only*. Once the protruded posture has become a habit and is maintained most of the time, it may also cause distortion of the discs contained in the vertebral joints. At this stage *movements as well as positions* will produce pain. Neck problems, developed in this way, are the consequence of postural neglect. Poor neck posture is not the only cause of neck pain. It is, however, one of the main causes and the most troublesome perpetuating factor.

During sitting, the position of the low back strongly influences the posture of the neck. If the low back is allowed to slouch, it is impossible to sit with head and neck pulled backwards. You can easily try this out for yourself. Unfortunately, once we have been sitting in a certain position for a few minutes, our body sags and we end up sitting slouched with a rounded low back *and* protruded head and neck. For most people sitting for prolonged periods results in sitting with poor posture.

ENVIRONMENTAL FACTORS

The design of transportation, commercial and domestic seating only encourages our poor postural habits. Rarely do the chairs available give adequate support to low back and neck and, unless a conscious effort is made to sit correctly, we are forced to sit badly. For the neck, ideally the back of the chair should come up high enough so that we can rest our head against it, but this support is not always included. An exception are the seats manufactured for most airlines but, unfortunately, their head-supports push head and neck into the protruded position which causes our problems. It is a brave person indeed who risks sleeping in one of these seats, for on waking he may well have the old familiar pains in the neck.

When travelling by car, train, bus or plane we are often compelled to sit in the position dictated by the seats provided. It may be necessary for the driver of a car, bus or truck, especially in bad weather, to protrude head and neck in order to peer through the windscreen.

Furniture in offices and factories all over the world is designed equally poorly and, to make matters worse, not adapted to individual requirements. This is one of the reasons that so many people who have a sedentary occupation, and spend most of the day in a seated working position, develop low back and neck pain. Until furniture designers understand the requirements of the human frame and manufacture accordingly, we will continue to suffer from their neglect.

Finally, the design of domestic furniture is not any better. Unless your favorite lounge-chair is exceptional, you will have insufficient support in low back and neck and will continue to place strains on these areas when you relax for the evening. If your neck problems are aggravated by reading or watching television, it is unlikely that the contents of the book, newspaper or television programme is giving you a pain in the neck. The posture that you have adopted is the cause of the pain, and this posture depends to a large extent on the type of chair or support you use.

Although the poor design of furniture contributes to the development of neck problems, equal blame lies with the way in which we use this furniture. If we do not know how to sit correctly, even the best designed chairs will not prevent us from slouching. On the other hand, once we are educated in correct sitting, bad chairs will not have a big impact on our posture.

HOW TO MANAGE PROLONGED SITTING SITUATIONS

In order to *prevent the development of neck pain* due to prolonged poor sitting it is necessary to (1) sit correctly, and (2) interrupt the protruded head posture or prolonged neck bending at regular intervals. In order to *treat neck* pain resulting from poor posture other exercises may need to be performed besides the postural correction. In this chapter I will only discuss the exercises required to reduce postural stresses and obtain postural correction. The exercises for relief of pain and increase of function will be dealt with in the next chapter.

CORRECTION OF THE SITTING POSTURE

You may have been sitting slouched for many years without neck and shoulder pain. But once you have developed neck problems you must no longer sit in the old way, because this posture will only perpetuate the overstretching discussed previously.

If you are sitting slouched with the low back rounded, it is not possible to correct the posture of the neck. (*Fig. 3:2*) Therefore it is necessary to *first correct the posture of your low back.* How to assume and maintain the correct posture of the low back in sitting is described in *"Treat Your Own Back"* also by Robin McKenzie. For the purposes of this book, however, you must be fully aware of the following. The natural hollow, present in your low back while standing, must be maintained during sitting in order to sit correctly. (*Fig. 3:3*) To achieve this *the use of a lumbar roll is essential.* A lumbar roll is a specially designed support for your low back (*Fig. 3:4*). The roll should

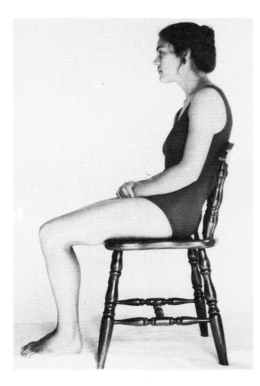

Fig. 3:2
Poor neck posture. The result of insufficient low back support.

Fig. 3:3
Good neck posture made possible with low back support.

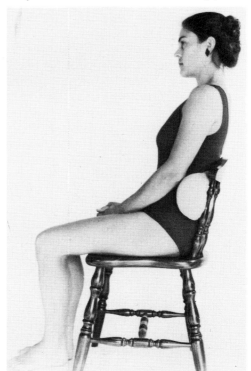

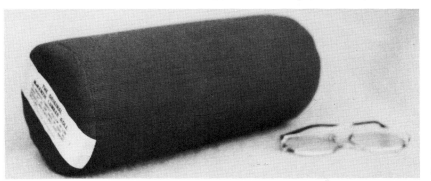

Fig. 3:4
Lumbar roll.

be no more than three to four inches in diameter before being compressed, and should be moderately filled with foam. Without this support your low back slouches and your head protrudes as soon as you relax or concentrate on anything other than your posture, for example when talking, reading, writing, watching television or driving the car. To counteract this slouching you must place a lumbar roll in the small of your back at the level of your beltline whenever you sit in an easy chair (*Fig. 3:5, 3:5a, 3:5b and 3:5c*), car (*Fig. 3:6 and 3:6a*) or office chair (*Fig. 3:7 and 3:7a*).

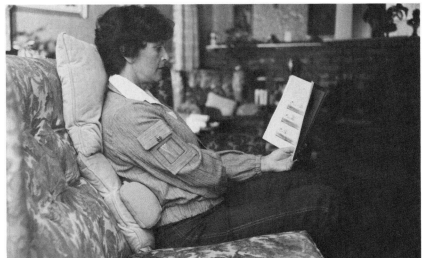

Fig. 3:5
Correct.

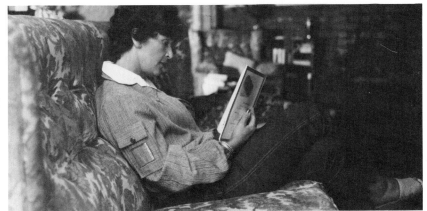

Fig. 3:5(a)
Incorrect.

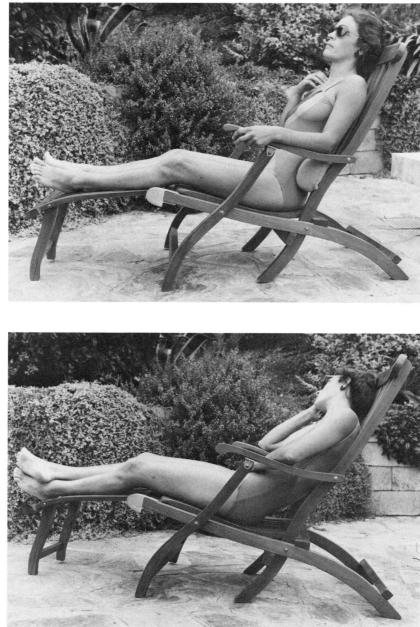

Fig. 3:5(b)
Correct.

Fig. 3:5(c)
Incorrect.

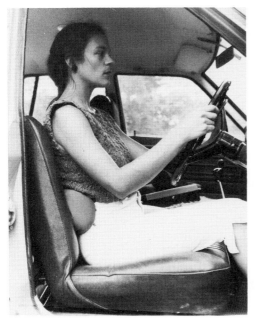

Fig. 3:6
Correct.

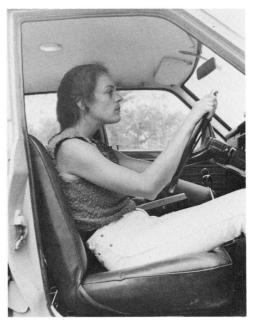

Fig. 3:6(a)
Incorrect.

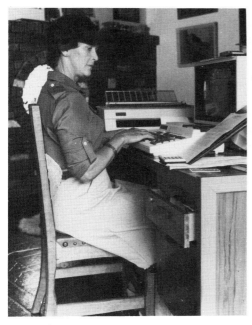

Fig. 3:7
Correct.

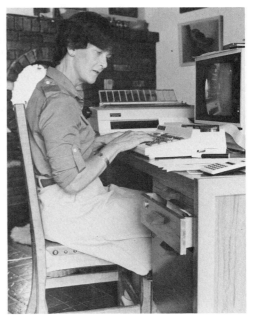

Fig. 3:7(a)
Incorrect.

In order to correct the posture of your neck while sitting you must first learn *how to retract the head.* Therefore you must become fully practised in Exercise 1 — head retraction (see chapter 4). This exercise should be performed fifteen to twenty times per session and the session should be repeated three times per day, preferably morning, noon and evening. The rhythmic procedure teaches you the correct position of your head in relation to the rest of your body. Each backward movement of the head must be performed to the maximum possible degree. When the head is pulled back as far as possible, you have assumed the so-called retracted head posture (*Fig. 3:8*). Now you have reached the extreme of the corrected head and neck posture.

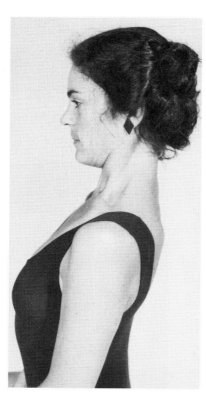

Fig. 3:8
Retract.

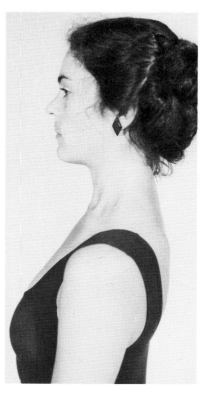

Fig. 3:9
Perfect correct posture.

Once you know how to retract the head, you must learn *how to find and maintain the correct head and neck posture.* The extreme of the retracted head position is a position of strain and it is not possible to sit in this way for a long time. To sit comfortably and correctly you must hold your head just short of the extreme retracted posture. To find this position you must first retract the head as far as possible (*Fig. 3:8*), then release the last ten percent of this movement (*Fig. 3:9*). Now you have reached the correct head and neck posture which can be maintained for any length of time. It may take up to eight days of practise to master this.

The aim of this part of the programme is to first restore the correct posture and then maintain it. As a rule the pain will decrease as your head posture improves and you will have no pain once you maintain the correct posture. The pain will readily recur in the first few weeks whenever you allow your head to protrude. But eventually you will remain completely painfree even when you accidentally forget your posture. However, you should never again allow yourself to sit slouched with a protruded head for a long time. As soon as you have been completely painfree for a couple of days, you can resume your normal activities. If from now on you follow the instructions given in this book, you may also be able to prevent further neck trouble.

When first commencing the above procedures to correct your low back and neck posture in sitting, you will experience some new pains. These may be different from your original pain and may be felt in another place. New pains are the result of performing new exercises and maintaining new positions. They should be expected and will wear off in a few days, provided postural correction is continued on a regular basis. Once you have become used to sitting correctly, you will enjoy it. You soon will notice the reduction or absence of pain and the increased comfort. From then on you will automatically choose chairs that allow you to sit correctly.

Rule: *When sitting for prolonged periods you must sit correctly with the low back supported by a lumbar roll and the head retracted.*

REGULAR INTERRUPTION OF PROLONGED NECK BENDING

If you spend long periods of time in the sitting position — for example while knitting or performing desk tasks —, it is likely that, even with the best of intentions, you will eventually forget to maintain the correct posture. Gradually you will assume a more or less protruded head posture or a position in which both head and neck are bent forwards. To counteract this you must frequently interrupt the forward bent position by correcting your neck posture and stretching head and neck backwards. (See Chapter 4. Exercise 2) This will relieve the stresses on the discs between the vertebrae as well as the surrounding tissues.

Rule: *When sitting for prolonged periods, regular interruption of prolonged neck bending is essential. This can be achieved by retracting the head and extending the neck five or six times at regular intervals, for example each hour.*

2. Lying and Resting

The next most frequent cause of neck pain is postural stress in the lying position. If you wake up in the morning with a stiff and painful neck that was not causing problems the night before, there is likely to be something wrong with the surface on which you are lying or the position in which you sleep. It is a comparatively easy task to correct the surface on which you are lying, but rather difficult to influence the position you adopt while sleeping. Once you are asleep you may just regularly change your position or you may toss and turn. Unless a certain position causes so much discomfort that it wakes you up, you have no real idea of the various positions you assume while sleeping.

CORRECTION OF SURFACE

All that is required to correct the surface on which you are lying is to alter your pillow. You may need to change the material of which it is made, the thickness of it, or both. You must realise that the main function of the pillow is to *support both head and neck*. Therefore it should fill the natural hollow in the contour of the neck between head and shoulder girdle without tilting the head or lifting it up. On the contrary, the head should be allowed to rest in a dish-shaped hollow. It follows that you must be able to adjust the contents of the pillow easily. Ideally your pillow should be made of feathers or kapok, with rubber or foam chips as a second choice. By pulling and pushing the contents you can make a hollow for your head and bunch the edge to form a thick support for your neck. Pillows made of moulded rubber or foam plastic do not allow their contents to be adjusted. They always adopt the shape or their original mould irrespective of attempts to change them. They do not permit the head to rest into a dish-shaped hollow but tend to apply a recoil pressure against the natural position the head would like to adopt. If you have such a pillow, you should replace it with one made of the recommended materials.

If, for some reason or other, the pillow does not provide adequate support for your neck, you should use a supportive roll in addition. Make a soft foam roll of about three inches

(8 cm) in diameter and eighteen inches (45 cm) long. (*Fig. 3:10*) Place this inside your pillow-case, on top of the pillow and along its lower border (*Fig. 3:11*). Alternatively, you can use a small hand towel of about twenty inches (50 cm) long and wide. Fold this in half and roll it loosely, then wind it around your neck and pin the ends together in front. In both cases the supportive roll will fill the space between pillow and neck. (*Fig. 3:11a*) The measurements, given above, are merely a guide. All neck supports need to fulfill individual requirements and each person needs to experiment for himself.

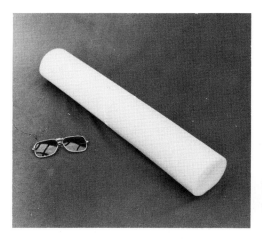

Fig. 3:10
Soft foam roll .

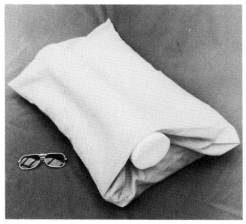

Fig. 3:11
. . . positioned inside pillow case.

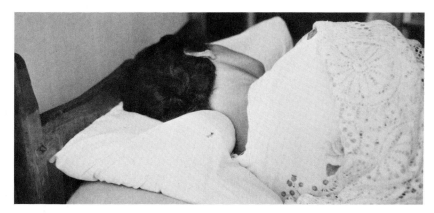

Fig. 3:11(a)
. . . in order to support the neck.

CORRECTION OF THE LYING POSTURE

If the lying posture itself is thought to cause the problems, it needs to be investigated for each person individually. But there is one position which requires further discussion. Some people like to sleep lying face down and frequently wake up with a pain in the neck or headache, which wears off as the day progresses. Other than this they seem to have no neck problems.

While lying face down the head is usually turned to one side and in this position some of the joints, especially in the upper neck, reach the maximum possible degree of turning or may come very close to it (*Fig. 3:12*). Consequently, this position places great strains on the soft tissues surrounding the joints of the neck and those between upper neck and head.

If you have problems of this nature, you must avoid lying face down. In addition it is advisable that you perform the recommended exercises, in particular exercises 1, 2 and 6 (see Chapter 4). This is to ensure that you can retract the head and extend the neck properly and have an adequate range of movement when turning the head.

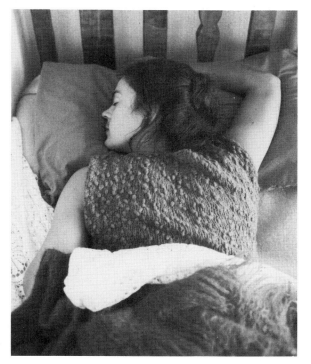

Fig. 3:12
This sleeping position causes excessive strain.

3. Relaxing After Vigorous Activity

When you have finished some vigorous activity — for example playing football or tennis or chopping wood — and have not suffered any pain as a result, *you should not relax by sitting or lying with the head in the protruded posture (Fig. 3:13 and 3:14)*. Thoroughly exercised joints of the spine easily distort if they are held in an overstretched position for prolonged periods. A commonly heard story is that a person, who sits down to rest following hard work, some time later has such severe pain that he can hardly move his neck. Usually people blame the actual activity as the cause of their trouble, but in most cases the pain is produced by prolonged forward bending of head and neck.

Rule: *After vigorous activity you should retract the head and extend the neck five or six times. If you sit down to rest, you should avoid the protruded head posture.*

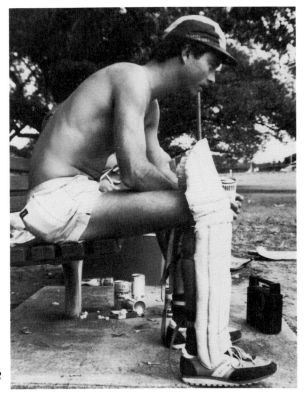

Fig. 3:13

4. Working in Awkward Positions or Cramped Spaces

Some jobs can only be performed in positions which are likely to cause overstretching of the neck. These jobs may require the adoption of the sitting position and usually they involve precision work. Alternatively, they may have to be performed in cramped spaces or with head and neck in awkward static positions. Under these circumstances you may not be able to prevent the onset of neck pain just by regularly assuming the correct posture. If your neck problems are brought on in this way, you must, in addition to postural correction, frequently interrupt overstretching and perform exercise 6 then exercises 1 and 2.

Rule: *When working with head and neck in a static position, you should at regular intervals interrupt this position by assuming the correct posture. In addition you should perform five or six movements of exercise 6, then exercise 1 and 2.*

Fig. 3:14

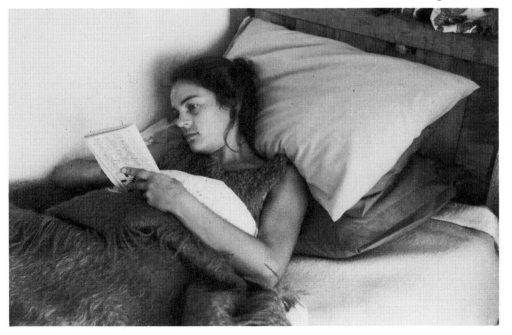

CHAPTER 4

EXERCISES

GENERAL GUIDELINES AND PRECAUTIONS

The purposes of the exercises are to abolish pain and, where appropriate, to restore normal function — that is, to regain full mobility in the neck or as much movement as possible under the given circumstances. When you are exercising for pain relief, you should move to the edge of the pain or just into the pain, then release the pressure and return to the starting position. But when you are exercising for stiffness, the exercises can be made more effective by using your hands and gently but firmly applying overpressure in order to obtain the maximum amount of movement. Postural correction and maintenance of the correct posture should always follow the exercises. Once you no longer have neck pain, good postural habits are essential to prevent the recurrence of neck problems.

In order to determine whether the exercise programme is good for you it is very important that you observe closely any changes in the location of the pain. You may notice that pain, originally felt to one side of the spine, across the shoulders or down the arm, moves towards the centre of your neck as a result of the exercises. In other words your pain localises or centralises. *Centralisation of pain (Fig. 4:1) that takes place as you exercise is a good sign.* If your pain moves from areas further away from the neck, where it is usually felt, towards the midline of the spine, you are exercising correctly and this exercise programme is the right one for you.

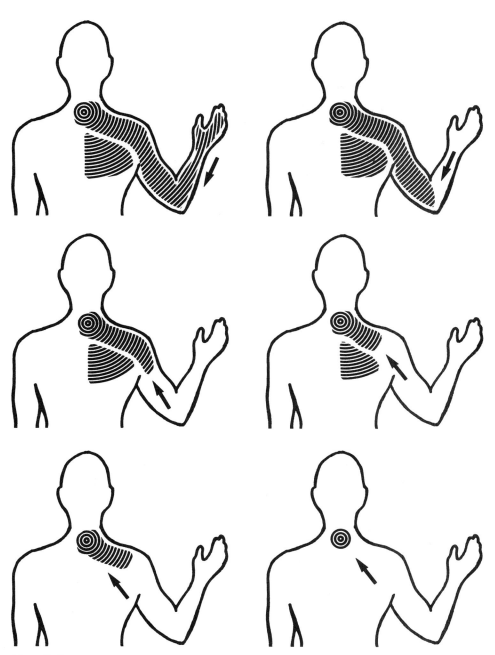

Fig. 4:1
Progression of centralisation of pain indicates suitability of exercise programme.

If your neck pain is of such intensity that you can only move your head with difficulty and cannot find a position to lie comfortably in bed, your approach to the exercises should be cautious and unhurried.

On commencing any of the exercises you may experience an increase in pain. This *initial pain increase* is common and can be expected. As you continue to practise, the pain should quickly diminish, at least to its former level. Usually this occurs during the first exercise session. This should then be followed by centralisation of pain. Once the pain no longer spreads outwards and is felt in the midline only, the intensity of the pain will decrease rapidly over a period of two to three days and in another three days the pain should disappear entirely.

If, following an initial pain increase, the pain continues to increase in intensity or spreads to places further away from the spine, you should stop exercising and seek advice. In other words, do not continue with any of the exercises, if your symptoms are *much worse immediately after exercising and remain worse the next day;* or if, during exercising, symptoms are *produced or increased in the arm below the elbow.*

If your symptoms have been present rather continuously for many weeks or months, you should not expect to be painfree in two to three days. The response will be slower but, if you are doing the correct exercises, it will only be a matter of ten to fourteen days before the pain subsides.

It is recommended that you adopt the sitting position when learning to perform the exercises. Once you fully master them you may exercise in sitting or standing, whichever is most suitable.

However, if the pain is too severe to tolerate the exercises in sitting, it may be necessary to commence exercising while lying down. In the lying position the pain will be reduced, because head and neck are better supported and the compressive forces on the spine are considerably less than in sitting. If you are sixty years of age or older, it is also advisable to commence exercising while lying down. People of the older age groups occasionally experience dizziness or light-headedness when performing extension exercises with the head. If these symptoms should persist you must stop the exercises and seek advice. On the other hand, when the initial attempts of extension exercises in lying do not have any ill effects, you can safely proceed to exercising in sitting.

If, due to some medical problems, it is difficult or not advisable for you to lie flat, you should restrict yourself to exercising in the upright sitting position.

When you commence this exercise programme you should stop any other exercises that you may have been shown elsewhere or happen to do regularly — for example for fitness or sport. If you want to continue with exercises other than the ones described in this book for neck problems, you should wait until your pains have subsided completely.

Once you have started this exercise programme, you should expect new pains to develop. These are different from your original pain and are usually felt in areas of the neck and shoulder girdle which were previously not affected. New pains are the result of performing movements your body is not used to and, provided you continue with the exercises, they will wear off in three to four days.

EXERCISE 1

Head Retraction in Sitting

Head retraction means pulling the head backwards. Sit on a chair, or stool, look straight ahead and allow yourself to relax completely. Your head will protrude a little as you do this (*Fig. 4:2*). Now you are ready to start the first and most important exercise.

Move your head slowly but steadily backwards until it is pulled back as far as you can manage (*Fig. 4:3*). It is important to *keep your chin tucked down and in* as you do this. In other words, you must remain looking straight ahead and should not tilt the head backwards as in looking up. When your head is pulled back as far as possible, you have assumed the retracted head posture (*Fig. 4:3*). Once you have maintained this position for a few seconds, you should relax and automatically your head and neck will protrude again (*Fig. 4:2*). Each time you repeat this movement cycle you must make sure that the backward movement of head and neck is performed to the *maximum possible degree*. The exercise can be made more effective by placing both hands on the chin and firmly pushing the head even further (*Photo 4:4*).

This exercise is used mainly in the treatment of neck pain. When used in the *treatment* of neck pain, the exercise should be repeated ten times per session and the sessions should be spread evenly six to eight times throughout the day. This means that you should repeat the sessions about every two hours. Should you experience severe pains on attempting this exercise, you must replace it with exercise 3. When used in the *prevention* of neck pain, the exercise should be repeated five or six times as often as required.

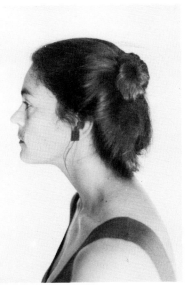

Fig. 4:2
The relaxed position allows
the head to protrude.

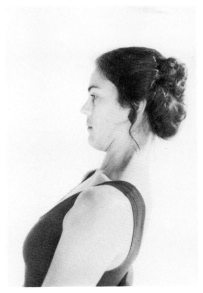

Fig. 4:3
The retracted position.

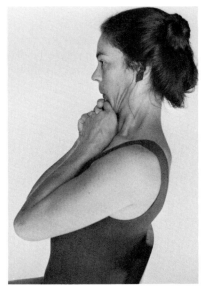

Fig. 4:4
Retracted with overpressure.

EXERCISE 2

Neck Extension in Sitting

Extension means bending backwards. This exercise should always follow exercise 1. Remain seated, repeat exercise 1 a few times, then hold your head in the retracted position (*Fig. 4:5*). Now you are ready to start exercise 2.

Lift your chin up and tilt your head backwards as in looking up at the sky (*Fig. 4:6*). *Do not allow your neck to move forwards* as you do this. With your head tilted back as far as possible you must repeatedly turn your nose just half an inch (about 2 cm) to the right and then to the left of the midline (*Fig. 4:7 and 4:7a*), all the time attempting to move head and neck even further backwards. Once you have done this for a few seconds, you should return your head to the starting position. Again, each time you repeat this movement cycle you must make sure that neck extension is performed to the maximum possible degree.

This exercise can be used both in the treatment and in the prevention of neck pain. Exercise 2 is to be performed ten times per session and the sessions should be spread evenly six to eight times per day. If your pain is too severe to tolerate exercise 2, you should replace it with exercise 3.

Once you are fully practised in exercises 1 and 2 separately, you can combine these two exercises successfully into one exercise.

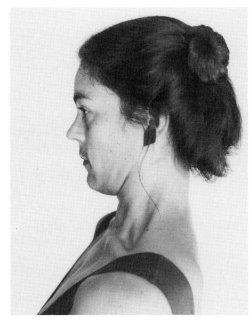

Fig. 4:5

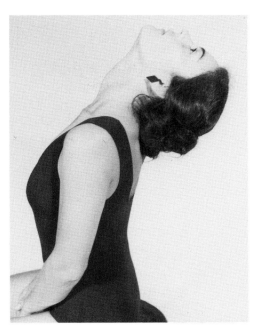

Fig. 4:6

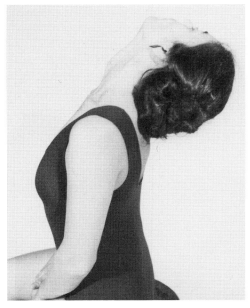

Fig. 4:7

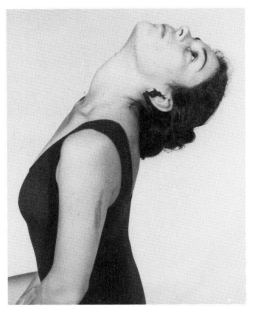

Fig. 4:7(a)

EXERCISE 3

Head Retraction in Lying

Lie face up with your head at a free standing edge of the bed — for example, lie across a double bed or with your head at the foot-end of a single bed. Rest head and shoulders flat on the bed and do not use a pillow (*Fig. 4:8*). Now you are ready to start exercise 3.

Push the back of your head into the mattress and at the same time pull your chin in (*Fig. 4:9*). The overall effect should be that your head and neck move backwards as far as possible while you keep facing the ceiling. Once you have maintained this position for a few seconds, you should relax and automatically head and neck will return to the starting position (*Fig. 4:8*). Each time you repeat this movement cycle you should make sure that the backward movement of head and neck is carried out to the maximum possible degree.

This exercise is used mainly in the treatment of severe neck pain. When you have completed ten head retractions, you must evaluate the effects of this exercise on the pain. If the pain has centralised or decreased in intensity, you can safely continue this procedure. In this case you should repeat the exercise ten times per session and spread the sessions evenly six to eight times throughout the day or night. But if the pain has increased considerably or extends further away from the spine, or if you have developed pins and needles or numbness in the fingers, then you must stop the exercise and seek advice.

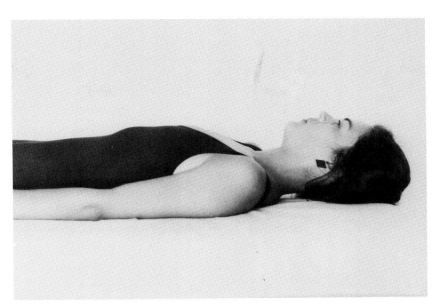

Fig. 4:8

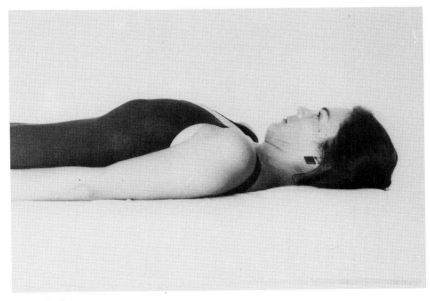

Fig. 4:9

EXERCISE 4

Neck Extension In Lying

This exercise should always follow exercise 3. Again you must lie face up on the bed. Before you can start exercise 4 you must place one hand under your head and move up along the bed until head, neck and the top of your shoulders are extended over the edge of the bed (*Fig. 4:10*).

While supporting your head you should lower it slowly towards the floor (*Fig. 4:11*). Now you remove your hand (*Fig. 4:12*) bring head and neck as far backwards as you can and try to see as much as possible of the floor directly under you. In this position you must repeatedly turn your nose just half an inch (about 2 cm) to the right and then to the left of the midline (*Fig. 4:13*), all the time attempting to move head and neck further backwards. Once you have reached the maximum amount of extension, you should try to relax in this position for about thirty seconds.

In order to return to the resting position you must first place one hand behind your head, then assist your head back to the horizontal position and move down along the bed until your head is lying on the bed again. It is important that, following this exercise, *you do not rise immediately* but rest for a few minutes with your head flat on the bed. *Do not use a pillow.*

As exercise 3, this exercise is used mainly in the treatment of severe neck pain. Until the acute symptoms have subsided exercise 4 is to follow exercise 3 and it should be done only once per session. Once you no longer have severe pains, exercises 3 and 4 should be replaced with exercises 1 and 2. By now you will have noticed that, except for the position in which they are performed, exercises 3 and 4 are really the same as exercises 1 and 2.

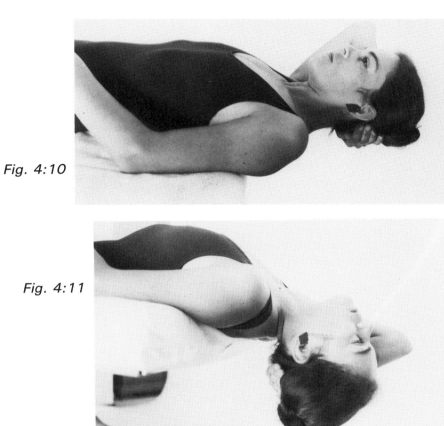

Fig. 4:10

Fig. 4:11

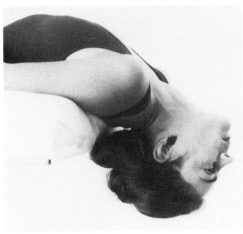

Fig. 4:12

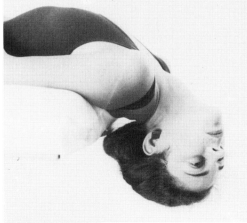

Fig. 4:13

49

EXERCISE 5

Sidebending of the Neck

Sit on a chair, repeat exercise 1 a few times, then hold your head in the retracted position (*Fig. 4:14*). Now you are ready to start exercise 5.

Bend your neck sideways and move your head towards the side on which you feel most of the pain. Do not allow the head to turn (*Fig. 4:15*). In other words, you should keep looking straight ahead and should not bring your nose but your ear close to the shoulder. It is important that you *keep the head well retracted as you do this. The exercise can be made more effective by using the hand of the painful side, placing it over the top of your head and gently but firmly pulling your head even further towards the painful side (Fig. 4:16).* Once you have maintained this position for a few seconds, you should return the head to the starting position.

This exercise is used specifically for the treatment of pain felt only to one side or pain felt much more to the one side than to the other. Until the symptoms have centralised exercise 5 is to be repeated ten times per session and the sessions are to be spread evenly six to eight times throughout the day.

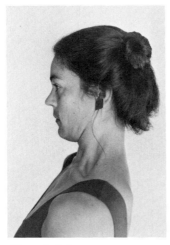

Fig. 4:14

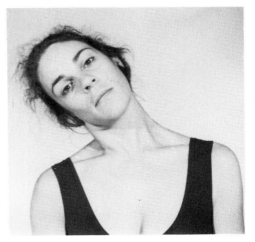

Fig. 4:15

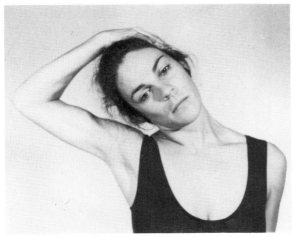

Fig. 4:16

51

EXERCISE 6

Neck Rotation

Rotation means turning to the right and left. Sit on a chair, repeat exercise 1 a few times, then hold your head in the retracted position (*Fig. 4:17*). Now you are ready to start exercise 6.

Turn your head far to the right and then far to the left as before crossing the street (*Fig. 4:18*). It is important that you *keep the head well retracted* as you do this. If you experience more pain on turning to the one side than to the other, you should continue to exercise by rotating to the most painful side and on repetition the pain should gradually centralise or decrease in intensity. However, should the pain increase and fail to centralise, you must continue to exercise by rotating to the least painful side. Once you have the same amount of pain or no pain but only stiffness when turning to either side, you should continue to exercise by rotating to both sides. The exercise can be made more effective by using both hands and gently but firmly pushing your head even further into rotation (*Fig. 4:19, 19a and 19b*). Once you have maintained the position of maximum rotation for a few seconds, you should return your head to the starting position.

This exercise can be used in the treatment as well as the prevention of neck pain. When used in the *treatment* of pain or stiffness of the neck, the exercise is to be performed ten times per session and the sessions are to be spread evenly six to eight times throughout the day. Whether centralisation or reduction of the pain has taken place or not, exercise 6 must always be followed by exercises 1 and 2. When used in the *prevention* of neck problems, the exercise should be repeated five or six times every once in a while or as often as required.

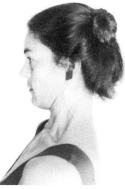

Fig. 4:17

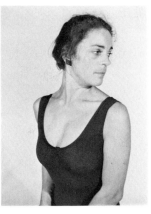

Fig. 4:18

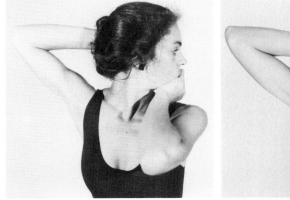

Fig. 4:19

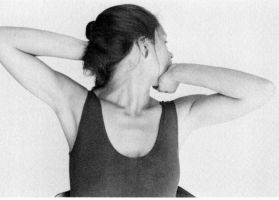

Fig. 4:19(a)

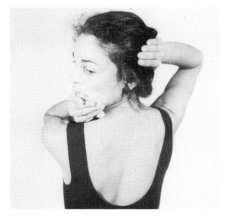

Fig. 4:19(b)

EXERCISE 7

Neck Flexion in Sitting

Flexion means bending forwards. Sit on a chair, look straight ahead and allow yourself to relax completely (*Fig. 4:20*). Now you are ready to start exercise 7.

Drop your head forwards and let it rest with the chin as close as possible to the chest (*Fig. 4:21*). Place your hands behind the back of your head and interlock your fingers (*Fig. 4:22*). Now let your arms relax so that the elbows point down towards the floor. In this position the weight of the arms will pull your head down further and bring your chin closer to the chest (*Fig. 4:23*). The exercise can be made more effective by using the hands and gently but firmly pulling your head onto the chest. Once you have maintained the position of maximum neck flexion for a few seconds, you should return your head to the starting position.

This exercise is used specifically for the treatment of headaches, but can also be applied to resolve residual neck pain or stiffness once the acute symptoms have subsided. In both cases it should be repeated only two or three times per session and the sessions should be spread evenly six to eight times throughout the day. When used in the treatment of headaches, exercise 7 should be performed in conjunction with exercise 1. When used in the treatment of neck pain or stiffness, exercise 7 must always be followed by exercises 1 and 2.

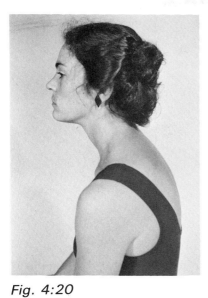

Fig. 4:20

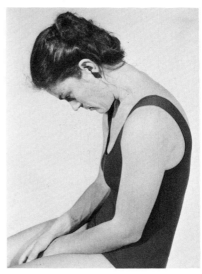

Fig. 4:21

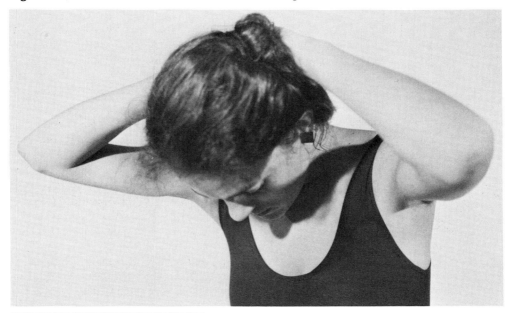

Fig. 4:22

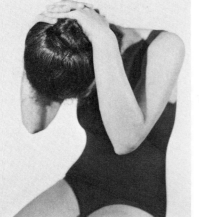

Fig. 4:23

CHAPTER 5

WHEN TO APPLY THE EXERCISES

WHEN YOU ARE IN SIGNIFICANT PAIN

If the pain is very severe, you may be able to get out of bed with difficulty, but certain movements will be impossible and often you cannot find a comfortable position in which to sit or work. Even though you have severe pain, you should always attempt to commence with exercise 1. Many people find that this exercise gives substantial relief from pain, and they do not have to start exercising in lying. As soon as possible, even on the first day, you should add exercise 2. You should continue the above exercises until you feel considerably better. Once you no longer have acute pain, you should follow the exercise programme as outlined for when acute pain has subsided.

If you have performed three or four sessions of exercise 1, spread over a period of fifteen minutes, and the pain remains too severe to tolerate this exercise, you should stop it and replace it with exercise 3. Your symptoms should gradually reduce and centralise so that there is some improvement by the time you have completed a few sessions. Exercise 4 should be added as soon as you have become well practised in exercise 3 and your symptoms have improved to some extent, or when you cease to improve with exercise 3. When to introduce exercise 4 varies from person to person, but the sooner you can do this the better. It is important that you carefully watch the pain pattern. You are exercising correctly, if in a few days the pain moves towards the base or the centre of the neck and decreases in intensity. In the end the pain should disappear entirely and be replaced by a feeling of strain or stiffness.

When you have improved significantly — usually two to three days after you commenced the exercises in lying, possibly earlier —, you may gradually reduce the number of sessions of exercises 3 and 4 and as you do this you should introduce and gradually increase exercises 1 and 2. In another few days you are only performing exercises in sitting and you will find that they give the same pain relief as you previously obtained by exercising in lying. At this stage the periods of time that you are completely free of pain are becoming more frequent and start to last longer.

Again, once you feel considerably better and no longer have acute pain, you should continue the exercise programme as outlined for when acute pain has subsided.

NO RESPONSE OR BENEFIT

When pain is felt only to one side of the spine or much more to the one side than to the other, the exercises recommended so far sometimes fail to bring relief. If this is the case, you should commence with exercise 5. Whether centralisation or reduction of the pain has taken place or not, exercise 5 must always be followed by exercises 1 and 2. After two or three days of practise you may notice that the pain is distributed more evenly across the spine or has centralised. Now you may gradually reduce exercise 5.

When you are considerably better and the pain has fully centralised, you should continue with the exercise programme as outlined for when acute pain has subsided.

WHEN ACUTE PAIN HAS SUBSIDED

Once the acute pain has passed, you may still feel some pain or stiffness when moving in certain ways. You will notice this best, when turning the head to the one or the other side or bending head and neck forwards to look down. It is likely that at this stage healing of overstretched or damaged soft tissues has taken place. Now you must ensure that the elasticity of these soft tissues and the flexibility of your spine as a whole are restored without causing further damage.

If you have pain on turning the head to the right or the left, you should practise exercise 6; and if you have pain on bending the head forwards, you need to practise exercise 7. Each time you repeat the exercise you must move to the edge of the pain and then release the pressure. The pain should disappear entirely over a period of two to three weeks. Each session of exercises 6 and 7 should always be concluded with a few repetitions of exercises 1 and 2.

If you feel stiffness only on these movements, you should do the same exercises but apply overpressure with your hands at the end of each movement. By exercising in this way you achieve movement to the maximum possible degree. In a period of three to six weeks you should be able to restore normal function.

Once you are completely symptom free, you should follow the guidelines given to prevent recurrence of neck problems. Now you should continue with the exercise programme as outlined for when you have no pain or stiffness.

WHEN YOU HAVE NO PAIN OR STIFFNESS

Many people with neck problems have lengthy spells in which they experience little or no pain. If, in the past or recently, you have had one or more episodes of neck pain, you should start the exercise programme even though you may be pain free at the moment. However, in this situation it is not necessary to do all the exercises and to exercise every two hours.

To prevent recurrence of neck problems you should perform exercise 6, followed by exercises 1 and 2 on a regular basis, preferably in the morning and at night. Furthermore, whenever you feel minor strain developing during work or while sitting, you should apply exercises 1 and 2. It is even more important that you watch your posture at all times and never again let postural stresses be the cause of neck pain. These exercises will have very little or no effect, if you constantly fall back into poor posture. It may be necessary to exercise in the manner described above for the rest of your life, but it is essential and imperative that you develop and maintain good postural habits.

As it takes only one minute to perform one session of exercise 6 and another minute to combine exercises 1 and 2 and repeat them ten times, lack of time should never be used as an excuse for not being able to do these exercises.

RECURRENCE

At the first sign of recurrence of neck pain you should immediately perform exercises 1 and 2. If your pain is already too severe to tolerate these exercises or if they fail to reduce the pain, you must quickly introduce exercises 3 and 4. If you have one-sided symptoms which do not centralise with any of these exercises, you should start with exercise 5. Again, you must pay extra attention to your posture, regularly perform postural correction and maintain the correct posture as much as you can.

WHEN YOU HAVE HEADACHES

Headaches can often be relieved by some of the recommended exercises, usually exercises 1 and 7. It will not do any harm to perform these exercises for a couple of days in order to find out whether you benefit from them or not. The first three days you should perform exercise 1 — head retraction — at regular intervals and whenever you feel a headache is developing. If this reduces your headaches but does not abolish them completely, you should add exercise 7. In particular the headaches which spread over the top of your head to above or behind the eyes are often relieved with this exercise. You may even be able to prevent the development of such headaches by performing this exercise as soon as you feel minor strain building up.

In case your headaches are not relieved by these two exercises, you should for the next three days do exercise 4 — neck extension in lying — followed by exercises 1 and 2 and postural correction. As your symptoms are improving you may gradually stop exercise 4 but you must continue with the other two exercises.

If you are unable to influence your headaches with any of the exercises or if your headaches become much worse during exercising and remain worse over the next day, you should stop exercising and seek advice.

CHAPTER 6
INSTRUCTIONS FOR PATIENTS WITH ACUTE NECK PAIN

Keep your head up at all times. When you allow the head to droop as in reading, knitting, sewing and performing desk tasks, you place further strains on the already overstretched or injured tissues. Maintenance of good posture is essential.

Do not roll the head around and avoid quick movements, especially turning the head quickly.

Avoid those positions and movements which initially caused your problems. You must allow some time for healing to take place.

Do not sleep with more pillows than necessary. If you are comfortable with one pillow, then use only one. The contents of the pillow should be adjustable in order to provide a proper support for the neck.

When you remain uncomfortable at night, you may benefit from a supportive roll.

Do not sleep face down, at this places great strains on the neck.

Do not lie in the bath for any length of time, as this bends your head and neck forwards, excessively.

Carefully start with the self-treatment exercises. Remember, an initial pain increase can be expected when commencing any of the exercises. This pain should reduce or centralise as you repeat the movements.

CHAPTER 7
SUMMARY

In order to treat present neck problems successfully you must do the following:

— **at all times**: correct your posture and maintain the correct posture.

— **when in acute pain**: if possible, perform exercises 1 and 2; if not possible, then do exercises 3 and 4.

— **when pain more to one side and not responding**: first exercise 5, later exercises 1 and 2.

— **when acute pain has subsided**: exercises 6 and 7, always followed by exercises 1 and 2.

In order to prevent future neck problems successfully you must do the following:

— **at all times**: maintain good postural habits.

— **when no pain or stiffness**: twice per day exercise 6, always followed by exercises 1 and 2.

— **at first sign of recurrence**: postural correction and exercises 1 and 2 at regular intervals — that is, ten times per session and six to eight sessions per day.

THE McKENZIE INSTITUTE INTERNATIONAL
SPINAL THERAPY AND REHABILITATION CENTRE
WELLINGTON, NEW ZEALAND

The McKenzie Institute International Spinal Therapy and Rehabilitation Centre has been established for the purposes of providing residential in-patient treatment programmes for patients with chronic and recurring back and neck problems.

The Centre accepts only patients whose symptoms have been present for three months or longer, who are experiencing significant disruption in lifestyle and who are unresponsive to usual outpatient treatment and who currently remain unimproved.

The Institute works directly with referring physicians and therapists in formulating individualised follow-up treatment programmes once the patient returns to the home environment.

If you would like more information about the Institute treatment programmes, please contact:

The Executive Director
The McKenzie Institute International
P.O. Box 93
Waikanae, New Zealand